GINSENG
'THE DIVINE HERB'

The Secrets of Chinese, Korean and Siberian Ginseng

Frena Bloomfield

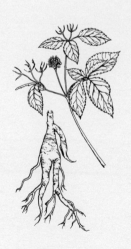

CENTURY
LONDON MELBOURNE AUCKLAND JOHANNESBURG

First published in 1987 by Century Hutchinson Ltd
62–65 Chandos Place,
London WC2N 4NW

Century Hutchinson Australia Pty Ltd
PO Box 496, 16–22 Church Street, Hawthorn,
Victoria 3122, Australia

Century Hutchinson New Zealand Limited
PO Box 40–086, Glenfield, Auckland 10, New Zealand

Century Hutchinson South Africa (Pty) Ltd
PO Box 337, Bergvlei, 2012 South Africa

Photoset by Deltatype Ltd, Ellesmere Port
Printed and bound in Great Britain by
The Guernsey Press Co. Ltd, Guernsey, Channel Islands

Additional research for this book was carried out by Gary Chak-kei Butt
and Mary Bernardi.

Are You Yin or Yang? and *Common Syndromes of the Major Organs*
tables are taken from *Harmony Rules* by Gary Butt and Frena Bloomfield
(Arrow, 1985)

British Library Cataloguing in Publication Data

Bloomfield, Frena
    Ginseng 'the divine herb' : the secrets
    of Chinese, Korean and Siberian ginseng. –
    (Miracle plants).
    1. Ginseng – Therapeutic use
    I. Title   II. Series
    615'.323687   RS165.G45

ISBN 0–7126–1543–1

I would like to dedicate this book to Michael Page instead of a letter.

Contents

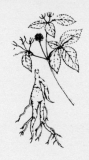

CHAPTER ONE
The Great Debate

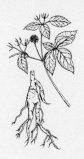

'Ginseng soothes base emotions, safeguards the soul, drives out fear, expels evil influences, brightens the eye, opens up the heart, increases the spirit and, if taken over a long period of time, prolongs life.'

So it was written in the *Shen Nung Pen Tsao*, China's first official pharmacopoeia, published almost 2,000 years ago, and it is still the way in which the uses and effects of ginseng would be described today by most traditional Chinese healers. However, until very recently, the attitude of the west towards ginseng could well have been summarised in the words of the writer who penned the article on ginseng in the last great scholarly edition of the *Encyclopaedia Britannica*. He concluded his article by writing: 'The action of the drug appears to be entirely psychic and compares to that of the mandrake of the Hebrews. There is no evidence that it possesses any pharmacological or therapeutic qualities.'

Even now, the popular opinion on ginseng is either that it is a miracle drug which cures all ills—as implied in its botanical name *Ginseng panax*—or, alternatively, that it is the botanical equivalent of the Indian rope-trick: an illusion experienced only by the credulous. The irony of both these views is that the Chinese, who until this century were the principal users of ginseng, have never claimed that the root was a miraculous cure-all. Meticulous to the point of being plain unimaginative, they carefully noted down throughout their 3,000 years of experience with ginseng its specific and general uses, together with strict guidelines about who should and should not use it. The greatest herbalist in China's history, the sixteenth-century master Li Shih-chen, would have been appalled by those who eagerly consume ginseng without regard to their body type and physical condition, just as he would have been puzzled by those self-styled experts who pronounced ginseng to be useless without ever having examined the properties and effects of the root. Two such experts were Dr Porter Smith and Dr Stuart, medical missionaries to China in the nineteenth century, who commented in their translation of Li Shih-chen's *Pen Tsao Kang Mu*: 'The ordinary ginseng of the market has been studied and has not been found to possess any important medical properties.'

To be fair, there are some very real barriers to be crossed when western medical science looks at Chinese medicine. The first and most obvious is that of language, but this is not a mere translation problem. It is also a historical and cultural problem. The terminology of Chinese medicine was established over 2,000 years ago and, on the whole, was standardised by about the fifth century AD. Ever since then, all new knowledge has been expressed in the same mystical Taoist language. This makes it particularly inaccessible to western medical experts who are already encumbered with a complex jargon of their own and are sometimes already predisposed to dismiss the medical knowledge of other cultures. A second major impediment is the essential difference in focus between Chinese and western medicine and the conditions they are intended to treat. Ever since the west turned from natural herbal medicine to chemical synthesis—now increasingly commercial interests are at work—western drugs have been aimed at very specific ailments, symptoms and conditions. However, Chinese medicine is entirely holistic and aims to return the whole body to balance. Thus, every symptom is seen as part of the whole and the pharmacopoeia reflects this too. The Chinese herbalist does not consider that isolating one specific element in the plant necessarily reflects its total therapeutic value and, in fact, traditional Chinese healers cite this bias in western medicine as being the cause of undesirable side-effects. However, this makes the task of the researcher—whether biochemist, physicist, botanist or doctor—very difficult when looking into the active factor in Chinese medicines. It can take years even to isolate the various elements, without starting on the task of conducting experiments and controls for a further period of time. On the whole, without the belief that he will indeed discover a usable and marketable drug, the researcher may well be understandably reluctant to undertake such a task. Promising young scientists cannot risk being stuck in an academic cul-de-sac.

However, during the past three decades, a number of factors have served to open up the investigation of ginseng with some exciting results so far and the promise of more to come. One is that there are now a significant number of Chinese scientists in the academic field. This has meant the entry into science of a group of people uniquely suited to investigate Chinese medicine. Already grounded in Chinese culture and language and also trained in western scientific method, they are able to bring together the oldest, most stable culture in the world and the newest scientific advances. Another encouraging factor has been the push from the World Health Organisation to investigate ethnic medical systems and discover whether there are valid herbal medicines which can be used to heal people and yet are free of both the side-effects and the prohibitive cost of western medicines. The other big push forward for ginseng came with a double accident of history—the occupation of Korea by Russia and the normalisation of political relations between China and the USA. The first brought Russia and consequently Russian scientists in contact with ginseng and the second brought western medical experts into the heart of the Chinese medical world, where both traditional and western medicine work together towards the one important goal— health.

The result of all this has been thirty years of scientific investigation into ginseng and its properties and effects. In Russia, Japan, Korea, Hong Kong, Switzerland and the USA, scientists have been making new and exciting discoveries about ginseng. The sixteenth-century herbalist Li Shih-chen described ginseng as being helpful in treating the following conditions: general debility, dyspepsia, fever and cold sweating, drowsiness and headaches, vomiting during pregnancy, apoplexy, malaria, internal injuries, sunstroke and internal bleeding. He also added that it increases vitality and prolongs life. So far, scientists have established that ginseng contains active ingredients which do the following: sedate and also stimulate when necessary, increase digestive function, reduce fatigue, reduce stress, stimulate the central nervous system, boost blood circulation, act in the same way as adrenaline, increase the synthesis of cholesterol, protect liver function, affect the endocrine system, and perhaps have a hormone-like effect. Further research is now looking into whether ginseng can control tumours, treat diabetes and act as an anti-ageing agent, since results now suggest that these are all possibilities.

It seems that the unlikely marriage of an ancient culture and a brash new school of knowledge has produced an entirely legitimate result—both agree that ginseng is a remarkable plant which has earned its ancient Chinese nickname of *shen tsao* or 'the divine herb'.

CHAPTER TWO
The Han People and the Earth Spirit

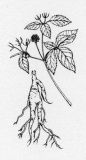

The Chinese claim to have been using ginseng for 5,000 years, but this is the legendary time period cited for the existence of every branch of the arts, crafts and sciences in China. It may possibly be a correct figure but we have no way of knowing that. Even so, it is certainly true that the Chinese have a long recorded involvement with ginseng and that written texts certainly take us back almost 3,000 years. Since it can reasonably be assumed that they experimented with the use of ginseng before they actually wrote about it and the first known reference appears in a manuscript from the third century BC, this suggests a respectably long acquaintanceship with the root.

The written reference appears in China's first official pharmacopoeia, *Shen Nung Pen Tsao*. This major collection of herbal knowledge and medical prescriptions is attributed to the legendary Emperor Shen Nung, hence its name. However, it is unlikely that Shen Nung was its actual author. Scholars still cannot be sure whether the early rulers of China who feature in popular folk-lore are legendary or historical figures. The two legendary rulers most often referred to are the Yellow Emperor Huang Ti and Shen Nung, known as the Holy Farmer. The Yellow Emperor is credited with writing *The Yellow Emperor's Classic of Internal Medicine*, the oldest medical textbook in the world and now dated to around 1000 BC by the latest scholarly estimates. Shen Nung is said to have died in the year 2698 BC and he is credited with inventing the lunar calendar by which China ran all its affairs until the setting up of the Republic in 1911. It was Shen Nung, so the story goes, who first classified all the plants according to their healing and medicinal qualities. The legend claims that he tasted over 170 herbs and roots, poisoning himself several times during this heroic task. It is undoubtedly because he was so closely associated in the popular mind with herbal knowledge that the first pharmacopoeia bore his name. All traditional Chinese scholarship is based upon attribution to past masters, in order to establish its pedigree and to show that it is firmly based upon established knowledge. Once this has been done, then the writer can include his own discoveries in the field. An additional factor is that many of the great teachings were passed down orally from master to pupil and it is entirely possible that the *Shen Nung Pen Tsao* was based upon a body of these oral teachings. They may indeed have come down from the legendary Shen Nung himself, if he ever existed.

It is this first official pharmacopoeia which contains the references to the virtues of ginseng that head the first chapter of this book. Since the reader may well be unfamiliar with the terminology of Chinese medicine, it is worth looking at that list of virtues and interpreting them, since they are not nearly as vague as they may appear to be at first glance. Taking it phrase by phrase, we shall see how the root is considered to work upon the body.

'Ginseng soothes the base emotions.' The seat of anger and impulsive drives is considered to be the liver, therefore ginseng works upon liver function. 'It safeguards the soul.' The soul or *shen* is centred in the heart, therefore ginseng improves the function of the heart and blood circulation. 'It drives out fear.' Fear is linked with the kidneys and impaired kidney function is said to underlie a fearful nature, therefore ginseng stimulates and improves kidney function. 'It expels evil influences.' The general term evil influences usually refers to diseases which are brought about by exposure to cold conditions, such as body aches and pains, muscular contractions, diarrhoea, nausea, indigestion and influenza. Ginseng counteracts these conditions and also generally increases the temperature of the body. 'It brightens the eyes.' In Chinese medicine, the eyes are associated with liver function and this is further reference to the fact that ginseng is considered to improve liver function. 'It opens up the heart and increases the spirit.' This is further reference to ginseng's ability to improve the function of the heart and increase energy.

Therefore, in the *Shen Nung Pen Tsao*, ginseng is recommended for use in improving the functions of liver, heart and kidneys and its regular use is considered to increase whole body vitality and to prolong life.

After the *Shen Nung Pen Tsao*, an increasing number of references appear in Chinese texts dealing with the medicinal or herbal aspects of ginseng, the difficulties of obtaining the root, or even its historical and political significance. The most prized ginseng of all was wild mountain ginseng which could be found rarely in the most remote mountainous regions of China. Therefore, an alternative source of supply had to be found. Conveniently, it was discovered to grow in Korea, which was a vassal state of the mighty empire of China. Ginseng roots were given as imperial offerings at least 92 times, and China opened a flourishing ginseng trade with the kingdom of Koguryo, the forerunner of modern Korea. In general, Korean ginseng was recognised to be greatly superior to most of the ginseng growing in China, with the exception of the rare wild mountain ginseng. In ancient times the best of this was said to come from the area of Shansi Province known as Shang Tang, although there is no ginseng there any more. The wild mountain ginseng was known as *Kung Bun*, which meant that it was solely for the use of the Emperor and his immediate court. All such ginseng automatically belonged to the Emperor, just as all swans in Britain belong to the reigning monarch. This, of course, did not mean that some of the precious root did not find its way into non-imperial hands, but it did mean that it was phenomenally expensive when it did. Wild mountain ginseng was prized because its properties were said to be so much more powerful than that of any other kind; the Emperor either used it himself or gave it to his immediate family or to high-ranking officials whose poor health was preventing them from carrying out their duties effectively.

The second medical reference to ginseng comes in a text written by a doctor who is virtually the Hippocrates of China, Chang Chung-ching (AD 142–220), known in his time as the Medical Sage and famed as a teacher. He wrote several classic medical texts, including *Attacked by Cold* which is still in print and used as a reference work by traditional Chinese healers. It is a study of the various illnesses caused by exposure to cold. He refers to his various experiments with ginseng and includes 21 prescriptions for its use. Some two centuries later, another famous herbalist, Ta'o Hung-ching (AD 452–536), revised the second edition of the *Shen Nung Pen Tsao* and later wrote a herbal of his own, known as *Ming I Pieh Lu*, to which he added many new prescriptions and included the first detailed botanical description of ginseng.

Because Ta'o was the first to describe ginseng in this way, a number of scholars have suggested that some of the early references to ginseng do not in fact refer to the plant now botanically labelled *Ginseng panax*. This is a view particularly held by Korean experts, but it is disputed by Doctor Paul But, one of the world's foremost botanical experts in Chinese medicines. He has considered the other plants put forward by scholars and says that they do not have the same properties ascribed to the ginseng root in old Chinese texts. Therefore, he is quite confident that the root identified in old Chinese pharmacological texts is the same as the one identified today as *Ginseng panax*.

In these early writings, a variety of names was used to refer to ginseng, some of them nicknames and some of them references to its uses. Among these were the following:

Gwei kai literally means 'ghost umbrella' and is a pun on the fact that the ginseng plant grows in the shadow of a tree and away from the touch of direct sunlight;

Shen tsao means 'divine herb';

Hsueh shen and *hong shen* mean 'yellow root' and 'red root'. These are not really just references to colour but to the doctrine of signatures which predominates in the Chinese pharmacopoeia. This also used to be a feature of the old European system of herbal lore and it is based upon the premise that like treats like—a simple example of this would be the treating of liver ailments by eating liver. However, it does become much more complicated than that and these two names refer to the assumption in Chinese medicine that yellow is associated with the spleen and red with the heart and blood vessels. Therefore, the yellower ginseng root is thought to be particularly good for treating the spleen and the redder root is especially good for stimulating the functions of the heart and the circulatory system.

Tu ching means 'earth spirit', a name derived from an old folk-tale reported to have originated in Shang Tang, in the following somewhat curious way. The Chinese had a passion for recording everything, which is why their written accounts of history, philosophy, the arts and every branch of knowledge, are so extensive. Records from all over China were collected by the Mandarins whose duty it was to administer the sprawling empire. These were the annals of the various imperial reigns. This story comes from the annals of the Sui Dynasty (AD 581–601), in the Shang Tang district, from which the best wild mountain ginseng came at that time. It was said that one night the inhabitants of a certain village heard a man crying in the darkness. All night long his voice could be heard from somewhere outside the village itself, begging and pleading. Next night, the same thing happened—a man could be heard calling pitifully all night long. The villagers were very frightened by this, being simple people and somewhat afraid of outsiders. Nevertheless, after the crying had gone on for several nights, a party of them got together and set off in the darkness to look for the source of the voice. About a mile from their village, they came upon the place where the voice was loudest. Seeing nothing which would account for it, they began to dig just where the voice appeared to be coming out of the ground. They cleared the earth away to a depth of five feet and there, lying in the ground in the exact shape of a man, was a huge ginseng root. It was this which had been crying out to be taken from the earth and henceforth the ginseng root was often referred to as the earth spirit.

Most commonly, then as now, the ginseng root is known among the Chinese as *jin shen* or 'man root', from its slight resemblance to the shape of a human form. In line with the doctrine of signatures, because of this resemblance, ginseng is assumed to be particularly good for treating human beings.

Chinese herbalists working through many centuries did not seem to vary greatly in their opinions about the properties of ginseng. From the first pharmacopoeia in the third century BC up to the herbal written by Ta'o Hung-ching in the fifth century AD, there were only a few effective additions made, namely that ginseng was to be used in treating thirst and polyuria due to diabetes, in reducing swelling and inflammation and was helpful in increasing the powers of the memory.

Among all these great men of learning, the one who towered over all the rest when it came to the Chinese pharmacopoeia was Li Shih-chen. In AD 1552 he took upon himself the task of compiling a great work which would incorporate all the knowledge contained in the thousand volumes which comprised the herbals of China. The result of this massive effort was the *Pen Tsao Kang Mu*, a 52-volume work which was completed by Li's son after his death and published for the first time in 1578. It is still in print today and is regarded as essential reading for all traditional Chinese healers. The work lists not only all the ingredients used in medical treatment—herbs, roots, minerals and animal products too—but also over 8,000 prescriptions.

Two American medical missionaries to China translated Li's *Pen Tsao Kang Mu* in the nineteenth century, adding explanatory notes and comments of their own. The Chinese, they noted, used five kinds of ginseng altogether, four of which were not derived from *Ginseng panax* at all. The other four were *sha shen*, or *adenophora*, which acted on the lungs; *hsuan shen* or *scrophularia*, which acted on the kidneys; *mou-meng* or *polygomum bistorta*, which acted on the liver; and *tan shen* or *salvia multirrhiza*, which acted on the heart. They also made mention of the classic test of whether a root was actually ginseng or not, a procedure which is still used today when there is doubt about genuineness of the root. Two people walk a mile together at a fast pace, each one with a small piece of ginseng in his mouth. If one of them reaches his destination faltering and out of breath, the root is not real ginseng.

Because ginseng was so highly valued in China, it was often given as a present, and in these instances the root was certainly Korean ginseng. Another medical missionary who worked in China during the nineteeth century wrote about this practice. 'In such cases, accompanying the medicine is usually given a small beautifully-finished kettle, in which the ginseng is prepared. The inner kettle is made of silver and, between this and the outer vessel, which is a copper jacket, is a small place for holding water.' The missionary was shown some choice ginseng by a herbal dealer who kept the precious root wrapped in silken cloth which was placed inside a silk-covered box. This in turn was kept inside a larger box lined with sheets of lead and all of this was packed round with little parcels of quicklime, to ensure that no moisture reached the dried root.

Today, even outside China, the Chinese form the bulk of ginseng buyers. This is demonstrated by the trade figures from Korea which show that the greatest amounts of the root go to Hong Kong and from there into Thailand, Indonesia, Taiwan and Singapore, as well as China itself. However, ginseng consumption is rising steadily in the west. In the USA, for example, there are estimated to be over six million users of ginseng, a large percentage of whom are not ethnic Chinese. However, the story of the west's involvement with ginseng was and is a complicated one which deserves a chapter of its own.

CHAPTER THREE
Ginseng and the West

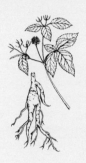

The west has had a longer involvement with the ginseng root than most people are aware of, but the relationship has been confused and complex. A number of factors have contributed to this situation. One is that for several centuries the west was not aware that there was more than one variety of ginseng and that the one used by the Chinese—*Ginseng panax*—had different properties from the other varieties which were all carelessly designated ginseng. This was a particular problem when it came to so-called American ginseng or *Panax quinquefolium* which, although a member of the same family, has sedating properties where those of the real ginseng are stimulating. This led to western medical and herbal experts dismissing some of the claims that the Chinese made for ginseng, unaware that they were not referring to the same plant. While the Chinese were fully aware of the different properties of the plants, the west was not.

That the west has now become equally aware of the special properties of ginseng is largely due to advances in science itself. Since the 1950s biochemistry has had the capacity to examine and isolate the active ingredients of the ginseng plant in a way that was not previously possible. Medical experts have tested ginseng extensively and there now exists a convincing body of research and experimentation which suggests that indeed ginseng may well have many of the properties that the Chinese have always believed that it has. Indeed, a number of current scientific investigations are beginning to suggest that some of ginseng's properties are unique.

So this century is seeing an end of the apparent clash between the ancient east and modern west and both are coming closer together in some agreement over the ginseng plant. It was after all back in AD 1000 that Ibn Cordoba brought back the first ginseng root to Spain, fruit of trading connections between the Arabs and the Chinese which had already existed for centuries. In fact, Arab physicians had taken a keen interest in Chinese medicine which they read in translation. During the first few centuries after the birth of Christ, Arab medicine was far in advance of that of Europe and the physicians of Arabia were much impressed by those of China. It was through this Arab interest that the art of taking the pulse was introduced into western medicine. However, the Chinese use it as an advanced diagnostic tool. They take the pulse at three points on each wrist, each one giving detailed information on the condition of a major organ of the body and the ailments affecting it. In this way, they obtain information which the western doctor can only extract through extensive laboratory testing. However, although the Arabs introduced the method into Europe, it has only survived as a simple heart-beat count.

From the time that Ibn Cordoba arrived with his ginseng specimen, Europe maintained a somewhat spasmodic interest in the root, although it was an interest in which fantasy played a strong part—this is probably still true when the rumours which surround ginseng's power as an aphrodisiac are considered. Marco Polo was the next to comment upon the plant, although historical opinion is divided about whether he actually brought any back with him. Certainly he found it in frequent use in China and noted this in his travel journals of 1294. He wrote: '[Ginseng] is powdered, cooked and used as a syrup or food, condiment, or even burned as incense in the sickroom.' He would have been aware of the importance of ginseng; at that time, it was already designated the imperial plant and was sold for its weight in silver.

Over the next two centuries, ginseng came to Europe largely through the agency of the mariners who were out prospecting for spices and colonies in the Far East. In 1610, for example, a Dutch sailor brought some back from his voyages. Another Dutchman, Hendrick Hamel, had the misfortune to be shipwrecked on an island off the coast of Korea in 1653, and was detained there until 1666, giving him plenty of time to gather material for his subsequent account of his travels—*Account of the Shipwreck of a*

Dutch Vessel on the Coast of the Island of Quelpart. Hamel mentioned that the cultivation of the ginseng root was a well-established practice in Korea.

However, it was in the eighteenth century that ginseng came to the fore in both Europe and North America and the catalyst which set the interest burning was a letter from China. The letter was written by a Jesuit missionary, an expert on topography and map-making who had been sent by the Vatican to the Emperor of China at his imperial request. This was Father Pierre Jartroux (1669–1720) who, on 12 April 1711, wrote a letter from Peking to his superior in Rome, the Procurator-General of the Mission for India and China. The letter was published by the Royal Society in London in 1714 and it is interesting enough to be quoted in full.

I wish the peace of the Lord be with you. In accordance with the order of the Emperor of China, we are making a survey to make a map of the Tartarian area. I acquired the opportunity to see the famous plant ginseng, which is not so well known to Europe but which is precious here in China. In July, 1709, we arrived at a village named Calca where Tartarians were living in the vicinity of 40 *li* from the Chosen Kingdom [Korea]. One man among us bought four pieces of ginseng root in a basket that they picked from the nearby mountains. I am sending a detailed sketch of one root to you. The explanation of the picture will be given at the end of this letter. Great medical scholars in China write many books about the effects of ginseng medicine.

Ginseng is added to almost all medicines for the nobles. Since the price of ginseng is too high, common people can hardly think of taking it as a medicine. Ginseng is a superior medicine for the fatigue caused by overwork of the mind and body. It is demulcent, alterative, tonic, stimulant and carminative, it strengthens the lungs and pleura, stops vomiting, increases the appetite, strengthens the function of the stomach, decreases the rush of blood, has the effect of curing giddiness, and prolongs the lives of old people. If ginseng had no such effect, Chinese or Tartarian people would never think so highly of the roots of ginseng. Even healthy people use ginseng internally to become healthier. According to my judgment, I believe that ginseng may become a wonderful medicine if it ever gets into the hands of European people who know about medicine and they make a study of various capabilities of ginseng by experimentation and chemical methods and conduct clinical tests for the actual diseases.

Undoubtedly, ginseng stimulates the circulation of the blood and heats the body, helps the function of digestion, and notably increases vigour. I was able to feel a remarkable strengthening of pulse when I measured my pulse one hour after taking half a root of raw ginseng. Appetite increased and more vigour resulted. The dexterity was improved after the intake. However, I suspected that such effects might have been brought by the rest. Similar effects occurred every time I took ginseng roots. But, four days later, I was exhausted from my work and barely able to endure sitting on a horse. A governmental employee who noticed such things by sense gave me one root of ginseng. I ate half the ginseng on the spot and fatigue disappeared completely one hour later. After this experience, I often ate ginseng. Same effects happened all the time. I was able to recognise the same effects when I chewed the fresh leaves. As Tartarian people did, I boiled ginseng into a medicinal tea. It has a good colour. You will know it has a good flavour too, when you drink it a couple of times.

If ginseng could be produced in any places other than Chosen [Korea], it would be Canada, for, according to a report by the people who once inhabited Canada, the forests and mountains of Canada are similar to those of Tartary. Tartarians call ginseng *Orhoda*, which means the best of all plants. There are enough reasons for this.

Father Jartroux wrote his letter at a time when there was already considerable curiosity growing in Europe about this root whose properties were mainly the subject of rumour. Then, as now, the mysterious east was credited with more than it claimed for itself—people thought that ginseng was the plant form of the alchemical Elixir of Life. They had heard vaguely, and supplied the rest from their own imaginations, that ginseng kept human beings young, kept them alive indefinitely and, best of all, kept men sexually potent beyond their wildest ambitions for themselves. It was stories such as these that kept excitement burning about the ginseng root. The Academy of Science in Paris had already made the use of ginseng as an aphrodisiac the subject of a learned discussion held in 1697. Following this, the French King, Louis XIV, had ordered his medical advisors to search out the plant wherever they could and, in 1704, one of them was able triumphantly to send some ginseng samples from Quebec in Canada. It was tried out as an aphrodisiac and apparently was not well-reported upon, but this is really hardly surprising since it was not *Ginseng panax* at all, but the sedating *Panax quinquefolium* which would have had more or less the opposite effect. This was the first time that the west started inextricably to mix up the two plants, erroneously believing that they had the same properties; this was the start of two centuries of confusion.

The aphrodisiacal fortunes of King Louis began to look up again when, in 1613, an ambassador sent to the French court by the King of Siam offered the French monarch his choice of rare and precious gifts, including ginseng roots. Naturally, his majesty chose the ginseng and, presumably having reported more favourably on its effects, a craze for ginseng possessed the aristocracy thereafter. It was at this point that Father Jartroux's much publicised letter began to bring results which were to open a whole new trade between the west and China.

Intrigued by Father Jartroux's suggestion that ginseng might be found growing in Canada, Father François Lafiteau, a French missionary who was administering to the faithful in the French colony of Quebec, took the drawing of ginseng that Jartroux had appended to his letter and showed it to some Mohawk Indians. They instantly recognised the plant and went off to find some samples of it for the priest. What they actually returned with was *Panax quinquefolium* but Father Lafiteau sent it off to Europe with the triumphant certainty that what he had found was oriental ginseng. It was the start of the ginseng trade between North America and China.

European merchants and traders were delighted by the reports that ginseng had been found growing in plenty all over the mountainous woodlands of Canada. Since there was still a passion for the root in Europe and everyone had heard about the fabulous prices the Chinese were prepared to pay for the ginseng root, they were sure they were all set to make their fortunes twice over. Every merchant who could began to commission consignments of the root from Canada, for sale in France and for re-export to the Far East, and the great ginseng hunt began which within a few years was virtually to strip Canada clean of the plant. While the chase was on, however, every Indian who thought he knew where to find it—and most of them were very skilled in herbal lore—was off on the trail of the shy elusive root.

Like the Chinese, the Indians were familiar with their own version of the ginseng plant and used it medicinally. They were not as enthusiastic about it as the Chinese, but then, although at that point neither realised it, they were not dealing with the same plant. Nevertheless, it was used in a variety of ways which differed slightly from tribe to tribe. The Mohawks used it as a general remedy without any specific application. The Penobscots considered it to be useful in cases of female infertility and made a tea from it by steeping the root in water. The Cherokees employed it as a headache remedy and applied it in cases of cramp and for women's gynaecological disorders. The Creeks drank it as an infusion useful for shortness of breath, infantile croup and fever. They also used it, as did the Alabama Indians, as a dressing for wounds. They cut the root and rubbed the resulting sticky sap on the open flesh. The Houmas boiled the root and made a tea for the treatment of vomiting, while the Potawatomis pounded the root into a soft pulp to make a poultice useful in cases of earache. They also soaked this pulp and made a wash for inflamed eyes.

Most of the early settlers from Europe were equally impressed with the medicinal virtues of what has now come to be called American ginseng, although they were undoubtedly influenced by what they heard from Europe about the real ginseng and assumed those same virtues to be present in their home-grown cousin-root. In some ways, a few of them resented Europe's passion for ginseng since it intruded into their lives in odd ways. As one of them grumbled, 'the Indians were so taken up with this business that the French farmers were not able during that time to hire a single Indian as they commonly do so to help them during the harvest.' Instead, the Indians were off tracking in the woodlands, searching for the profitable root which merchants were eager to ship off to Europe.

The Indians were not the only ones who were out searching in the woodlands—so too were those settlers who had become convinced of the healing properties of the plant. William Byrd of Westover noted in his diary: 'The Root of this is wonderful Vertue in many cases, particularly to raise the Spirits and promote Perspiration.' He reported finding some American ginseng growing in the woods: 'I carry'd home this Treasure, with as much Joy as if every Root had been the Graft of the Tree of Life, and wash't and dry'd it carefully.'

In response to the general excitement about ginseng, most herbalists in Europe had by then at least obtained a sample of the precious root for their stock, even though they might not have been actually using it very much. Of course, there is no way now of knowing whether the root carried by the European herbalists was of *Ginseng panax* or of American ginseng, but they used them both for the same ailments and conditions. In general, herbalists used it for stomach ailments and nervous disorders for which both plants would have been effective. In Holland, herbalists were using ginseng regularly by 1736 to treat exhaustion and general debility and by 1741 it had been included in the official pharmacopoeia of Wurttemburg for treatment of similar conditions. In 1750, a great surgeon and botanist of the day, Albrecht von Haller, recommended the use of ginseng for treating gastric ailments and loss of memory.

By the 1770s, there was a steady trade in the export of American ginseng from Canada and America. The first shipment which had gone from Quebec to Canton in 1720 had been a failure. The Chinese found that the root which had been sold to them as ginseng was nothing of the sort, but a lookalike interloper with few of the same properties. However, detailed experimentation with this new plant soon revealed that it had virtues of its own which had medicinal uses. Its main property was that, contrary to real ginseng, it was a cooling or sedating root. Once the Chinese had incorporated this into their pharmacopoeia they were willing to continue buying it, although it was never highly valued and its price reflected this. Nevertheless, those who were involved in the export of American ginseng still made trading fortunes with the root, buying it cheaply from the Indian hunters and selling it by the ton to China. Their trade figures for those years reflect the value of the export business; in 1773, for example, the American ship *Higham* carried 55 tons of American ginseng to Hong Kong for shipment into China. In 1784, another American ship, *The Empress of China*, bore 40 tons to Canton. The trade continued unabated for the next 150 years, reaching its height in the early years of this century. In 1906, for example, the USA exported 160,940 tons of the root to China.

The trade contained the seeds of its own destruction. The ginseng hunters of North America had nothing in common with those of China. For one thing, they were ignorant of the plant and had little idea that its value depended upon its age. They just looked for a ginseng plant and hauled it out of the ground. The idea of leaving it to mature and be useful for another generation far in the future would have been laughable to them had it ever crossed their minds. The results of this were that Canada was stripped clean of ginseng within a few years and that America has followed the same path. Now, the trade is not worth even half a million dollars a year at a time when a single good root of the best ginseng can fetch US$100,000.

The United States' official pharmacopoeia included American ginseng in its listings from 1842 to 1882, but put it into the secondary list. By 1883, it was dropped altogether and is never likely to return since the pharmacopoeia includes drugs which are specifics and not ones with the multi-faceted properties that ginseng seems to possess. For many years, western experts regarded ginseng—both American and *Ginseng panax*—as a root which had been credited with powers only by uninformed and superstitious people and it is possible that this state of affairs would have continued were it not for accidents of war and peace in this century: principally the occupation of Korea by the Russians, the normalisation of the relationship between the USA and China, and the invasion and subsequent occupation of Korea by the Japanese for the decade from 1930 to 1940. During this period of time, the Japanese observed and took a great interest in the growing of ginseng. The centuries of trade between Korea and China had long since made it obvious to the Koreans that they would have to grow ginseng on a domestic basis instead of relying upon finding it growing naturally. The ancient and most valuable kind of ginseng, wild mountain roots, was as rare in Korea as it was in China. Therefore, they had set up ginseng plantations in which the plants were raised for use both within Korea and for the export trade in which they were a major item. The Japanese centralised control of the ginseng growers and nationalised their production, bringing everything under state control as it remains today.

Korea suffered a second occupation, this time by the Russians, between 1945 and 1948. They were equally intrigued by ginseng and Soviet scientists started to study the plant extensively, while the adminstrative officers devised a plan for growing ginseng in Russia. They carried out this scheme with such success that by 1958 they had set up a nursery of some 60,000 ginseng plants seized from Korea. Even before this, however, Soviet scientists had begun working on ginseng and Professor Israel Brekhman, after more than a decade of research, published the results of his own study of ginseng in 1957. Most of the latest studies in ginseng have come from Russia and Japan, a side-effect of war.

The other big factor in changing the west's perspective on ginseng was the normalisation of relations between the USA, and therefore the west, and China. This has allowed many western observers to visit China, a number of whom have had a particular interest in medicine and healing. China has offered them an insight into healing that is unique. Due to necessity and the 3,000-year history of its own school of medicine, China was not inclined to jettison that knowledge, firmly based as it was upon so many centuries of practical experience. At the same time, neither was China about to refuse the new medical knowledge of the west, particularly in those areas where development has been slow—surgery and antibiotics especially. Therefore, what China has is something entirely of its own: country-wide medical care which offers both western and Chinese medical practice side by side. Thus, those first visitors to communist China were astounded to see modern surgical techniques being carried out while a patient remained fully conscious under the anaesthesia of acupuncture needles. They found that the Chinese had long ago discovered the use of natural ephedrine for the treatment of asthma, seaweed with its iron content for treatment of goitre, the use of natural insulin for those with damaged pancreatic function. There are many more medicinal advances newly-arrived in the west, yet already centuries-old in China. Moreover, the Chinese seemed to be working both systems with no apparent problem about accepting both. Intensely pragmatic people, they were obviously only interested in what was effective. This gave westerners the chance to see Chinese medicine at work and started to raise questions for them which had never been entertained before. It suggested that, when it came to healing, the Chinese knew what they were doing at least as well as the west did and in certain instances somewhat better, although they were also always ready to learn new and better techniques from others.

Thanks to these various developments and to the entry of a number of Chinese scientists into the field of research—in China itself, in the USA and in Hong Kong—the secrets of ginseng are now being revealed in a way which is acceptable to the scientific establishment of the west, and can be explained in a way which western readers can comprehend.

CHAPTER FOUR
Ginseng and Chinese Medicine

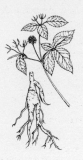

Because the only really extensive information that exists on the use of ginseng comes to us from the realm of Chinese medicine, in order to understand the guidelines it gives us it is necessary to understand a little about the basic principles of Chinese medicine. The first and most important point is that it is entirely holistic, treating the whole body system with the aim of returning it to harmony. Therefore, it does not treat individual symptoms but a whole syndrome in its particular human context. Just as each disease is unique, so is each person and the traditional Chinese healer will consider both before beginning his treatment.

There are a number of complex philosophical concepts which underlie Chinese medicine, of which the chief is that of yin and yang. According to the Chinese, everything in the universe is either yin or yang, even down to the tiniest particle. Yin and yang are an indivisible pair which together create balance. They are never fixed, since there is nothing in the physical world which is not in constant motion. As atoms and molecules are constantly on the move, so too is the balance of yin and yang constantly changing. Everything has a small measure of the both yin and yang in it, just as the man has a small element of the female hormone in him, just as the woman has her measure of the male hormone. This is just a living example of the yin-yang principle at work. The same principle applies to everything medical. The

Are You Yin or Yang?

Characteristic	Yin	Yang
Typical behaviour	introverted, easily tired, sleeps curled up, often closes eyes, prefers the shade, suffers from depression, often looks sad or worried, over-controlled	excitable, restless, irritable, active, eyes wide open and alert, stretches frequently
Physique	slightly built, weak, movements lack energy	large build, strong, energetic
Complexion	pale, sallow but occasionally with red spots on the cheeks	red-faced, blushes easily, eyes often inflamed
Body temperature	low, often has cold hands and feet, tendency to run a low temperature in the afternoons	warm skin, hands and feet, easily develops fevers
Sensitivities	enjoys massage, often has numbness or dull pains in the body, itchiness	gets severe stabbing pains, hot flushes, dislikes massage, burning sensations in the body
Muscle tone	weak flabby muscles, little flesh	muscular, tense muscles, very active
Respiration	weak, shallow, often short of breath	heavy breathing, tight chest
Eating pattern	poor appetite, suffers indigestion, likes warm food and drink	good appetite, excellent digestion, likes cold food and drink
Bowels	soft stools, tendency to diarrhoea, undigested food passed in stools	constipation, hard stools, burning sensation in the anus
Urination	frequent, can lose control of urination, clear in colour	infrequent, difficulty in passing urine, yellow in colour
Sweating	cold, light	hot or no sweating at all
Menstruation	blood light in colour, often late, small flow, pain after period is over	dark heavy flow, often clotted, usually early or less than 28-day cycle, pain before flow starts
Palpation of abdomen	soft, feels no discomfort	hard, tense, painful
Tongue	pale, dilated, covered with thin white coating, insensitive	red, dry, solid-looking, thick coating, very sensitive
Pulse	weak, slow	strong, fast

Common Syndromes of the Major Organs

Heart:

Symptoms	Tongue	Pulse
Deficient		
quiet in mien, palpitations, shortness of breath, fatigue, cold sweat, tight chest, poor memory, facial oedema, numbness in the extremities	dilated pale tongue with thin white coating	small, weak, missed beat
Excess		
insomnia, irritability, chest pain, palpitations, fever delirium, stroke, neurosis, thirst, bitter taste in the mouth, pain in the tongue	red, dry	large, strong, fast, irregular

Small intestine:

Symptoms	Tongue	Pulse
Deficient		
abdominal pain, cold sweat, cold feeling in the abdomen, diarrhoea, indigestion	pale, feels tender, thin white coating	small, weak, slow
Excess		
restless, blood in urine, sluggish urination, pain in the penis, distension of abdomen, flatulence	red, dry, yellow coating	smooth, fast

Liver:

Symptoms	Tongue	Pulse
Deficient		
poor vision, dizziness, numbness in muscles and tendons, pain in scrotum, hernia pain, nervous insomnia, palpitations	blueish, white coating, wet	deep, tight, slow, weak
Excess		
red painful eyes, restlessness, irritability, thirst, bitter taste in the mouth, dark yellow urine, dizziness, migraine, pain in the ribs, numbness in fingers, ringing in the ears, tremors, cramps, restless in sleep	red, dry, yellow coating, tremor	tight, fast, strong

body's organs are yin or yang, its functions are yin or yang, even its diseases are yin or yang—and both yin and yang are in constant flux. The yin-yang table [see page 29] will supply further examples of each.

In terms of Chinese medicine, yang usually refers to conditions which over-stress the functions of the body. The kind of conditions which are considered yang include inflammation, strokes, heart attacks, high-stress conditions like ulcers, and cancers, and in general anything which comes on suddenly and acutely. Yin conditions would include all that indicates the under-functioning of the body, like anaemia, diarrhoea, nervous breakdowns, breathing problems, impotence and indigestion, among others. All chronic and longterm conditions which are not life-threatening but are difficult to cure are yin.

Another way in which the terms of yin and yang can be expressed in Chinese medicine is that yin can be regarded as cooling or deficient, while yang is heating or excess. As both these terms are unclear to the westerner, it is probably better to say that yin means sedating and yang means stimulating, especially when applied to medicines. One of the things a Chinese healer will do before prescribing medicines is to consider all aspects of the case—and then decide if the system essentially needs calming down or stimulating. As a further guide for the reader, the tables showing the common syndromes of the major organs [see page 30] will help to demonstrate what the doctor may be looking for in his examination. The one major aspect of Chinese medicine which is confusing to westerners is that the names which are given to illnesses and medical conditions in the west are merely regarded as metaphors by the Chinese doctor. It is difficult for us to realise that the same disease may be entirely differently described in another culture and entirely differently treated, although the end result may well be the same cure. For example, what we call a heart attack would be a disease of yang excess to the Chinese doctor and he would give equal importance to all the accompanying symptoms; the cold sweating which goes with the pain, the muscular cramps, the dizziness, the ringing in the ears, the breathing difficulties. He would be looking for a herbal medicine which would work on all of these symptoms simultaneously and harmoniously. He would not be looking for something to sedate only the heart, especially if it were at the cost of suppressing other functions which actually needed stimulating.

A disease can change the nature of the patient by affecting his natural inclination to be either yin or yang. For example, we can see this in the person with hepatitis who becomes irritable and short-tempered even though normally he is quiet and calm in temperament. In Chinese medical terms, his usual yin nature is overpowered by the yang excess of the disease—hepatitis, being an inflammation, is yang—and it temporarily makes him behave in a yang excess manner. The doctor would be looking for a treatment which calms down the over-excited liver and consequently brings the patient back to his balanced self.

Another important idea in Chinese medicine is that all the body's organs produce their own energy, called *chi*. Each organ has its own measure of this. Heart *chi* controls the function of the heart and the circulation of the blood, lung *chi* controls breathing and the circulation of oxygen in the body, and so on. This *chi* is regarded as being in flux and it can be increased by the correct medical treatment and diminished by disease and bad living. If, however, its measure falls below that at which it can maintain the function of the organ and below the point at which it can be further stimulated by any kind of treatment, death will result. There is only one exception to all of this and that involves the kidneys. According to Chinese medicine, the kidneys have a number of functions. They not only control the excretion of water from the body, but are also associated with growth and with sexual function. Sexual energy is derived from kidney *chi*. In addition to this, life *chi* is also seated in the kidneys. Life *chi* comes from the parents. It is the human being's hereditary energy for life itself and it is not renewable. It cannot be increased by medical treatment but it can be diminished by the wrong sort of living. Therefore, the forces of life, growth and sexual energy all centre on the kidneys.

Chinese medicine works much more slowly than western medicine. This means that it does not on the whole have the capacity to move quickly against emergency conditions, for example those requiring the heavy use of antibiotics. Also, since there were historical and cultural bans on the dissection of the dead, surgery was not highly developed among the Chinese and their anatomical knowledge is still in some ways hazy. However, Chinese medicine's great virtue is that it works without the invasive and sometimes dire measures that accompany western medicine. It works by restoring balance to the whole and this is the aim of all Chinese medical treatment, including that which involves the use of ginseng.

When it comes to applying this to ginseng, the healer, of course, takes into account the nature of ginseng itself. Since everything is either yin or yang, so too are the medicines. *Ginseng panax* is very yang and therefore it is used for treating the conditions that require such properties. The information in this chapter comes from one of Hong Kong's most famous herbalists, Kwan Pak-cheung, now in his seventies. Mr Kwan is from a family renowned as the biggest herbal medicine dealers in southern China, with their main warehouse sited on the city of Canton. When he was a young man, he was educated at the College of Traditional Medicine in Canton, which was considered to be one of the foremost traditional medical schools in the whole of China. He has been a practising herbal doctor for 50 years and is regarded as an expert in the use of ginseng.

In Chinese medicine, there are ten kinds of ginseng in common use, all but one of them *Ginseng panax*, but which vary greatly in quality and effect.

Wild mountain ginseng is the choicest of all and comes now only from the Manchurian mountain areas. The ginseng hunters search for the root on the forested slopes of the mountains, looking for the Kia tree under which the plant likes to shelter. They only pluck the root if it is between 80 and 100 years old. If it is younger, they leave it for another time or even another generation to pick. This ginseng is regarded as being of unparalleled power, both because of its extreme age and also because of the untramelled purity of the environment in which it grows. It is so powerful that it is reputed to continue affecting the body for a year and it is also this plant which is said to keep the dying alive at least for the three or four days it takes to get the family together around the bedside. That was one of the uses of the plant in earlier times and, in fact, Mr Kwan has an example of this from his own family. It occurred when he was a young man.

He said: 'When my sister was about to get married, the bridegroom's mother fell seriously ill and it was obvious that she was going to die. Her one wish was to live just long enough to see her son married, so my family decided to help. We gave her 9 grammes of the finest wild mountain ginseng from our herbal store and made it into a tea which she could drink. Well, she drank it and she lived seven days more, enough to see the wedding safely over. But then, because of the power of the plant, she couldn't die and she was suffering terribly. Our family made another tea for her, this time of the Chinese radish which has the effect of neutralising ginseng and at last she died peacefully.'

As might be imagined, this precious root is not cheap. The current price is around £100,000 for one ounce. One of the reasons for this is that only twenty pounds of the root are found in an entire year and most of it is kept for the use of China's leaders—which may well be one reason why they seem to live to such an active old age. For the very small amount which comes out of China there is a waiting list of a year and most of the root is snapped up eagerly by Chinese millionaires wanting to preserve all those powers which made them rich in the first place. Since the root is so expensive, it has never so far been investigated in the same way as other younger ginseng roots. Few scientists have big enough grants to pay out the price but just recently in Hong Kong an American scientist bought roots to the value of US$500,000 for research purposes, so we may see interesting new data appearing over the next few years on this particular kind of ginseng. In the meantime, we have to go by the guidance of the herbalist who says that the active ingredients of ginseng increase in their power as they age. Science has nothing direct to say about this, but significant implications have emerged through experiments. Ginseng must be over three years old before its active ingredients begin to develop. Whether they continue to develop for the next 100 years western science cannot yet tell us. It seems reasonable to assume that Chinese medical experts may well have been on track once more with their own experiences of using the ancient root over the centuries.

Korean ginseng is now virtually all grown on special plantations as part of the national control of production. *Tin* means sky or heaven and it describes the best Korean root. In appearance it is a very solid root which, when sliced, has rings inside somewhat like those of a tree. It is called red ginseng but actually it is dirty brown in colour.

The second quality Korean ginseng is called *dei*, which means ground, and this root is not so solid looking. In fact, when sliced it usually has hollow cavities inside it. Both the Korean ginsengs are considered to be the best commercially available root and they cost over £1,000 an ounce for the best and around £800 an ounce for the second quality. The therapeutic effects last for about a month.

There are six kinds of Chinese ginseng in common use by herbalists—*sek chiu sum* (stone pillar ginseng), *dai ji sum* (prince ginseng), *soung ching sum, ching dong sum, lou dong sum*, and *yuen sum*. These all come from northern China and are of increasingly lower quality, their effects lasting for barely one week. *Soung ching sum* has the power to tone *chi*, which means that it generally stimulates the energy of the whole body system. *Ching dong sum* is thought of as toning the heart: it stimulates the heart and makes it work more efficiently. *Yuen sum* is considered to tone *chi* but at the same time to sedate the function of the lungs. Each of these roots fetches only about £100 for a pound, which demonstrates its therapeutic value as far as the Chinese are concerned. They are the roots that the poor would have to make do with.

American ginseng, the one which caused all that confusion in the west, is a member of the same family but not the same plant. Its botanical name is *Panax quinquefolium* and Chinese herbalists regard it as having different qualities from ginseng proper. There is a school of thought in herbalism that, just as poisonous herbs and their antidotes are thought to grow near each other, in the same way the herbs that people need grow in their own country. Chinese people need toning because their natural inclination is to be yin. In more accessible medical terms, they suffer from slow debilitating conditions and frequently tend to be somewhat neurasthenic and nervous. David Bonavia describes this well in his excellent book, *The Chinese*, by commentating that the Chinese have a very high boiling point but are troubled by an undercurrent of hysteria in their general makeup. These, of course, are generalisations but they indicate that the need is there for a strong strengthening tonic such as ginseng. On the other hand, westerners in general are regarded as being very yang. They are outgoing, individualistic, stressed, place a low value on serenity and harmony, preferring stimulation and are subject to conditions which erupt suddenly and powerfully when it comes to sickness, such as cancer, heart attacks and strokes. Therefore, they need calming down and their systems need cooling. Fortunately, American ginseng does just this. It sedates where ginseng proper stimulates. It draws heat from the body and in western terms this means that it lowers the stress level and eases tension. It is also regarded as being good for relieving drunkenness. American ginseng currently fetches around £300 per pound for farm-grown roots and around £500 for wild roots.

There is one other kind of ginseng which sometimes appears on the market. In Cantonese it is called *ak pei sum*, which means white skin ginseng, and it is actually American ginseng which had been taken and replanted in Japan. However, the replanting has caused peculiar problems. Putting the cooling American ginseng into Japanese soil, which is extremely sulphurous and full of phosphor, has turned it into a curious hybrid, a cooling plant which has become warming. It is regarded as an extremely poor-quality plant with limited properties of healing. It is the lowest grade available on the market.

Which brings us to the big question: what exactly does ginseng do? Is it the great aphrodisiac the west believed, and not only the west, if it comes to that? There are still plenty of Chinese around who think of it as an aphrodisiac. Does it prolong life? Is it a cure-all? In fact, western science now has some exciting answers for us on those questions, which we will come to in a later chapter. Meanwhile, the advice of the Chinese herbal expert is as follows:

'Ginseng is for people who need toning, for yin people. It can be useful for those who suffer from a lack of energy, from under-functioning organs. This is why it is so good for old people. The process of becoming old is a yin process and therefore the taking of ginseng increases the old person's yang and restores function. This is why we say it prolongs life in old people. It is excellent for the nervous system in people who are under-functioning. The legends about ginseng as an aphrodisiac are largely false. Now, if your sexual functioning is threatened because your kidneys are deficient, then ginseng will restore that ability. People who have sex a lot deplete the power of their kidneys and ginseng can certainly help restore this. This is probably how the stories started in the first place. But, no, it isn't an aphrodisiac. It cannot supply function where desire itself cannot.'

In western terms, the kind of conditions which are most responsive to the use of ginseng are low body temperature, low blood pressure, shortness of breath, chilliness and general debility. Westerners must be careful about taking ginseng. It should not be taken by yang types, so the yin-yang table should be consulted before you take it. If you are yin, you can take ginseng without danger. If you are yang, it can be dangerous. You should certainly not take ginseng if you think any of the following attributes describe you—if you have a red face, if your eyes are inflamed, if you are restless and irritable, if you have mouth ulcers, bright red lips, bad breath, burning indigestion. Any of these indicate that you are already in a heated condition and that to increase it would be foolish, if not actually dangerous. You should look instead to American ginseng.

If you disregarded the advice of the Chinese herbalist, you run the risk of showing some signs of ginseng abuse. Very little research has been done into this, but one study undertaken by the Department of Psychiatry and Biobehavioural Sciences, UCLA, indicates that hypertension, restlessness, insomnia and general nervousness result from such incidents. In Hong Kong itself, still the biggest consumer of ginseng, at least one hospital has reported several instances of what appears to be ginseng abuse which resulted in temporary paralysis of the eye muscles, causing a severe squint and double vision. A hospital stay of two or three days has usually seen the condition disappear with no further complications arising.

CHAPTER FIVE
Science and Ginseng

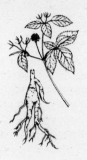

Ginseng has probably been the subject of more research in this century than any other plant in history. Although it was dismissed in the early years of the twentieth century as being only the focus of various native superstitions, the problem was not ginseng. The problem was that science itself had simply not progressed far enough for scientiests to investigate the true properties of the plant. With the tremendous advances in biochemistry that occurred from the 1950s onwards, it was possible to analyse the plant and to discover what it might be capable of doing. That research is still in progress all over the world but particularly in Russia, the USA, Japan and Korea, as well as in the country most involved with the history of ginseng—China.

Some of the most exciting research of all is going on in Hong Kong. The Chinese University of Hong Kong has a whole project devoted to the interdisciplinary study of ginseng and its proper-ties. This is actually part of a larger programme which is examining the entire pharmacopoeia of herbal material used in Chinese medicine, using the backing of IBM machinery and funded at least partly by the World Health Organisation. The research team consists of chemists, biochemists, botanists, zoologists, pharmacists, anatomists, physiologists and social scientists and, as well as carrying out their own investigations, they are also checking out more than 30,000 files of reports from

China where continuous western-style experiments have been carried out with ginseng. On the whole, most research has naturally enough been done by those countries which have a special investment in ginseng. These include Russia, which has grown ginseng since the 1950s and which has a native variety of plant popularly but incorrectly called Siberian ginseng, Korea, which is the world's main exporter of the plant, and China, which is the biggest user.

So far, research into ginseng has revealed that the plant contains a group of eighteen chemicals known as ginsenosides which are regarded as the most important active substances in the root. Since 1984, further substances thought to be of considerable importance have been isolated and these include an insulin-like protein and a possible anti-ageing agent known as maltol. There are also a number of polysaccharides, as well as various minerals, such as iron, and vitamins. The full chemical identity of ginseng has not yet been fully established and there is no doubt that more remains to be discovered. The complex nature of the specific chemicals in ginseng indicates that it will probably take years to complete these studies and the irony of it all is that science may well only end up confirming what that wise old Chinese herbalist wrote about its properties two thousand years ago.

Scientific research has already indicated that ginseng is involved in the following functions in the body:

It affects the circulatory system by demonstrating a marked cardiotonic action while also lowering blood pressure by affecting the muscles of the blood vessels.

It increases the production of red blood cells.

It controls hypoglycaemia by increasing the intestinal absorption of phosphorus and the synthesis of energy-rich compounds.

It affects the central nervous system in a non-specific way. In fact, experiments show that small amounts stimulate, while large amounts sedate.

Long-term usage increases physical and psychological efficiency without causing sleep disturbances.

It increases accuracy of work, concentration, and prevents fatigue.

Large doses have shown analgesic, anti-convulsant and anti-pyretic action.

It normalises liver function and may also decrease blood alcohol concentration.

It affects nucleic acid in the body, helping to maintain metabolic balance under stress.

It affects the endocrine system either by stimulating it or even by acting itself as a hormone—scientists are not sure which.

It stimulates the thyroid to normal action.

It stimulates the gonads, especially in older people.

It counteracts the problems caused by lack of testosterone.

It has an action prohibiting the growth of tumours which is still being debated and investigated.

However, the most remarkable property of all in ginseng is so exceptional that a special word was invented, by the Russians, to describe it. They called ginseng an adaptogen. An adaptogen is a substance which can act according to the needs of an organism and not according to its own fixed and immutable nature. It is a concept which is enough to cause heart attacks in those who are responsible for itemising the properties of a drug for marketing. Virtually all western drugs have only specific uses. In fact, it is impossible to register for medical use a drug which is not specific. This is why, for example, a plant with the healing properties of *aloe vera* cannot be an official remedy even though it is the best possible treatment for small burns and cuts. Ginseng, with its unique property of being an adaptogen, is a bureaucrat's nightmare and a scientist's dream. It is the reason why ginseng ever got its name in the first place; *Ginseng panax*, the panacea that cures all ills. It is not, of course, a panacea for all ills—no plant is—but it does cure a very varied list of ills, and others it helps very greatly. The power of ginseng is to normalise function where it is abnormal and it can be equally effective in, for example, both hypo- and hyperglycaemia.

The inference that can be drawn from the effectiveness of ginseng in such a wide variety of conditions is that it is most efficacious against conditions in which stress is the major precursor of imbalance and therefore of disease. Of course, it may well be—and increasingly is—argued that all illness is preceded by stress which enables breaches in the body's defence system to occur. However, this is still regarded as not proven by a number of medical authorities which link only certain diseases with stress. Among these are several heart conditions, hypertension, high blood pressure and a variety of symptoms like fatigue and tension. All of the effects mentioned above have come out of the wide variety of different experiments being carried out all over the world and much still remains to be done. Although there are many investigators, they are not working together in any organised way, and their experiments are often determined by differing sets of academic and investigative circumstances. Therefore there is no overview and no definitive conclusion available. This says as much about the present state of investigative science as about ginseng. The greater part of research of this kind is funded by drug companies' commercial ends, and it is virtually impossible for a non-specific like ginseng, which apparently has widely applicable and varied uses, to be marketable as an accepted drug. This limits the amount of research being done, since most researchers are working towards a product which will be commercially exploitable. It also makes it hard for western medicine to pronounce upon ginseng and indicate the ways it could be used by patients seeking to alleviate specific conditions. It is worth making these points since it is common for uninformed medical opinion to state that ginseng does not have any effective medical value or use. In fact, all experiments so far lead investigators to infer that it has many uses. The problem is to quantify them and ultimately to prescribe for them in a way that fits the western synthetic drug framework. We are simply not used to a wide-acting substance which treats a variety of apparently unlinked symptoms and conditions.

Apart from the individual investigations of ginseng in relationship to a wide variety of medical conditions, outlined above, its general properties are its ability to increase endurance and resistance, its anti-cancer possibilities and—one aspect which many consider the most exciting of all— its anti-ageing properties. Ginseng's ability to counteract fatigue has been widely investigated throughout the world, mainly in the USSR, Japan and Switzerland. The Russians particularly have carried out many experiments which show that ginseng increases performance and physical condition, and enhances mental capacity. The Russians were among the earliest scientific investigators of ginseng and their fullscale studies began back in the 1940s. This was partly because Russia has incorporated herbal medicines into the standard medical pharmacopoeia, for obvious practical reasons. The plants are widely available, they are a much cheaper source of usable and effective drugs than synthetics, and in the USSR there is not the same commercial pressure upon researchers to produce a synthetic which can be manufactured and marketed by a drug company seeking to get ahead of the competition. To a certain extent, we might conclude that a purer form of research may well be possible under such conditions.

The most famous name in Soviet research into ginseng, and one which comes up again and again, is that of Professor Israel Brekhman, now head of the Institute of Biologically Active Substances in Vladivostock, which is the Far Eastern branch of the Academy of Sciences of the USSR. In 1948, when Professor Brekhman was a young researcher, he carried out experiments in which he gave small amounts of ginseng to Russian soldiers who gave improved performances in various physical tests. Results like these have been reproduced many times over in other countries.

The problem for science is that it has many times recorded such results but without being able to agree exactly what it is that increases performance when the ginseng is absorbed. Other experiments have isolated so many ways in which ginseng does affect the body—through affecting the function of the liver, heart, endocrine, nervous and digestive systems—that this debate is not likely to end for a long time. The western investigative mode of reducing the whole to its tiniest parts is not ultimately as useful as the Chinese mode of observing the whole in action. In western terms, we shall have many more years to wait for the final word on ginseng. In Chinese terms, we had the information three thousand years ago.

Ginseng's properties as an adaptogen—a term devised by Brekhman and his associates to describe its ability to enhance function as necessary to affect the effects of stress—have also raised exciting questions in the use of the plant as an anti-ageing agent. The Chinese have a long tradition of believing that ginseng does keep the old young and the rich still pay happily to get hold of the best ginseng for this purpose—most usually expressed as maintaining sexual function, which is not a bad way of measuring the working capacity of the physical body, after all. It means more to most people than an eye test would do.

However, the Russians wanted to know more about the ways in which ginseng functioned and to do this they examined the ageing process. Most people are familiar with the outward effects of age but in this century in particular—and in youth-centred cultures like that of the USA this is of supreme importance—scientists and medical personnel have been asking what ageing really is and whether it is in fact as inevitable as we have thought in the past. One of the discoveries of the Soviet scientists was the use of ginseng against free radicals which are now thought to be the chief factor in physical ageing. A radical is normally part of a chemical grouping within a molecule, but it can break away from the group, becoming a free radical when the body is subject to various stress factors such as radiation or the taking in of certain kinds of food and drink, among other causes. Russian researchers have postulated that free radicals disrupt the normal processes of the body and set up adverse conditions that eventually lead to serious illness and the breakdown of function. Some researchers have concluded that many of the adverse factors in ageing are actually due to the accumulation of free radicals in the body and a number of experiments have confirmed that using ginseng does significantly reduce their destructive effects. The Chinese, through long centuries of using the plant, linked it with an anti-ageing effect which has now become legendary. Science is beginning to confirm the truth of the legend and it would not be too unlikely to assume that it will uncover many of the other truths about the plant which has been the subject of so much speculation and assertion in the past.

CHAPTER SIX
Siberian Ginseng

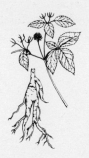

In recent years, a lot of excitement has been generated in the popular press about a plant usually referred to as Siberian ginseng. This name is not totally inaccurate—it does grow in Siberia—but that does not tell the whole story. The plant which has caused such a stir is actually more correctly known as *Eleutherococcus senticosus*, sometimes referred as Eleuthero for short. It is a member of the same family as *Ginseng panax*, the Araliaceae family, but it grows further afield than the Soviet Far East or Siberia; it can also be found in the same spartan terrain in Korea, Japan and China.

It became popular in Russia because of its association with the space programme and training regimen for Olympic athletes. That made it a big hit with the Soviet population in general, presumably because some of the glamour of the product was felt to rub off on somewhat more ordinary Soviet citizens. It is from these same connections that the western media suddenly became obsessed with this apparently newly-discovered miracle plant and a rash of articles has appeared in recent years making all kinds of claims for the plant and its ability to increase stamina and performance.

However, this is no new miracle plant. The Chinese, so often the first to make great discoveries, had already documented the existence of Eleuthero almost two thousand years ago. They called the plant *Ciwujia* (spelling varies but this is the generally used pinyin version of the Chinese name) and it is referred to in several of the early herbal pharmacopoeiae, including the *Pen Tsao Kang Mu* by China's greatest herbalist, Li Shih-chen.

There are also references to it in the first great herbal, *Pen Tsao* written in AD 200, but scholars are still arguing about whether or not this is the plant referred to now as Eleuthero, whereas they are mostly agreed about it in Li Shih-chen's herbal. It was and is a native of Heilongjiang Province and can be found growing in areas extending along the Xian Hinggan Ling Mountains. It has been studied extensively at the Heilongjiang Institute of Traditional Medicine, in Harbin. The Institute has hosted at least one international conference devoted to *Ciwujia* and regularly publishes reports about research into the plant and its properties. The Institute's most recent report on the plant indicates that it enhances the immunity of the organs to disease, promotes endocrinal function, regulates metabolism and also has been observed to have a certain curative effect on cardio-vascular and nervous diseases.

This ties in very well with the results of Russian investigations into Eleuthero. Most of the interest which has fired enthusiasm all over the world for this previously largely-unknown plant is due undoubtedly to the efforts of Professor Israel Brekhman, who had already previously researched ginseng (and also, incidentally, *Aloe vera*). While his investigations of *Ginseng panax* brought exciting results, there were problems. Little *Ginseng panax* grew in Soviet territories and much of that was in almost inaccessible areas and it is an expensive plant to consider buying, especially the better grades which might be assumed to have greater pharmaceutical properties. Therefore, he began to investigate the other members of the Araliaceae family which were known to grow in the USSR. One of these was Eleuthero and, since early results of his work looked promising, he continued to push on into the exploration of this particular member of the family. His first published reports began to appear in 1958 and they were so favourable that the Soviet government began clinical testing of the plant. It was this which started to attract attention to the plant, not only from members of the international community of scientists but even from the general public in Russia. It was only twenty years later that the west really started to pay any attention to this promising new rival of ginseng.

Widespread publication of the results of Brekhman's research into Eleuthero stirred academic interest all over the world and experimentation and testing has now been carried out—and still continues—in Europe and the United States of America, as well as in the Far East, including China. The most interesting discovery of all about Eleuthero is that it is what Brekhman describes as an adaptogen, like *Ginseng panax*, and it is its adaptogenic abilities which have attracted attention in the western press.

Not that it was necessarily the word used by media people. The articles which appeared in the west told mainly of how this miracle plant enabled people to work longer, better and harder, even people under extraordinarily stressful conditions such as astronauts—in a totally alien environment in which many detailed tasks have to be performed over and over again and from which there is no escape until they are brought back down to the earth's surface again. They told how Soviet athletes, recognised as probably some of the hardest trained in the world, could perform with more endurance and speed when helped by Eleuthero, which nevertheless did not in any way break the international regulations about drug use.

The promise was that, if it could do all that for those in extreme need, it could certainly do a great deal to make every day life more full, fun and faster-moving for everyone else. Indeed, scientific investigation shows that Eleuthero can do all that, but common sense should suggest that it cannot offset the ways in which people abuse their own bodies. Eleuthero enhances performance in a number of ways and it has brought about excellent results in treating a number of conditions—and basically that is that.

However, the news is exciting enough. Experiments have shown that people perform physical tasks better after taking Eleuthero for several days, and that some did better even when given only one dose soon before a race. It has been observed to increase people's visual and aural capacities. It has been established that it enhances resistance and restores haemoglobin levels in the blood. It has been used in the treatment of disease with some remarkable results.

Soviet scientists have observed that Eleuthero seems to have an inhibiting effect on tumours, as well as boosting the body's immune system. It reduced cholesterol levels in patients with arteriosclerosis as well as bringing about considerable improvement in their general condition—reducing confusion, controlling pain and bringing down blood pressure levels. It is effective in the treatment of diabetes and reduces blood sugar levels within an hour of ingestion. It has also been found to be helpful in treating radiation sickness by keeping down the number of white cells in the blood and raising levels of haemoglobin. Eleuthero has been tested upon patients suffering from nervous and neurasthenic disorders and seems to bring about more equable states of mind, reducing agitation.

It has been used in the treatment of a number of specific conditions, as the above indicates, but its great value—like that of *Ginseng panax*—is the way in which it enhances the whole performance of the physical system. It has a general mildly stimulating effect which increases functioning; hence its ability to reduce blood pressure and blood sugar levels. It regulates the endocrine system, reducing the effects of stress thereby. It regulates the cardio-vascular process, normalises the function of the central nervous system and has a stimulant effect on the sexual glands. It enhances immunity, as demonstrated in numerous Soviet experiments in which control groups showed a much higher rate of sickness and infection than the group regularly taking Eleuthero over extended periods.

Modern science is very ill-adapted to investigating a plant with properties as wide-based as Eleuthero. The problems are the same as those which bedevil the investigation of ginseng. The plants work on the whole system, bringing about increased harmony in the operational functions of the total organism. However, western science always takes things apart to find out one by one what the separate parts do. This makes a detailed investigation of the many properties of Eleuthero lengthy and costly. The investigation is still going on to find out why it works as it does.

The theory about Eleuthero is that its principal active ingredient is to be found in its glycosides, sugar-based compounds which have now been dubbed eleutherosides. Current investigation has established that there are 16 eleutherosides, 6 senticosides, isofraxidin, vitamin C, sucrose, beta-carotene, glucose, polysaccharide, vitamin E and traces of copper. Scientists think that the central mysteries of Eleuthero are contained in those 16 eleutherosides.

CHAPTER SEVEN

Treating Yourself with Ginseng and Eleuthero

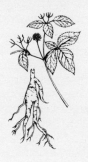

The first thing that any traditional Chinese doctor would tell you is to be sure you actually need to take *Ginseng panax*. Just because it is in itself a powerful tonic it does not necessarily mean you should take it. It depends upon your own state of health and whether or not you are in a yin or yang condition. As a general rule, many Chinese doctors would question whether a westerner needs to take ginseng. Many westerners are considered to be yang. That, say the Chinese doctors, is why so-called American ginseng—*Panax quinquefolium*—is a plant with many different properties from *Ginseng panax*. It is essentially a 'cooling' tonic—that is, it is a mild sedative, and it also improves general functioning. It is much more suitable for Americans, who tend to be yang rather than yin, and that is why it grows where it does.

Therefore, do not take ginseng just because it helps many Chinese people. The Chinese, in general, tend to be yin and need the yang boost of ginseng. Typical western conditions for which you could usefully take ginseng are low body temperature, low blood pressure, shortness of breath, chilliness and general debility, and how much you take depends upon the quality of the ginseng you buy.

This is the recipe suggested by Hong Kong's premier importer of ginseng, a millionaire many times over and considered to be one of the world's greatest experts on ginseng. Assuming you buy a good medium grade of Korean ginseng, take 9 grammes of the root and put it into an earthenware pot, together with 10 black dates from which the stones have been removed. Add 1 piece of fresh sliced ginger root and 2½ cups of warm water and simmer this mixture overnight. Drink it on an empty stomach first thing in the morning.

Remember that more is *not* better. It is possible to overdose on ginseng. You will not die of it but it overstretches the nervous system, making you feel taut and tense, which is the very opposite of the intended effect of ginseng. It can also elevate the heart beat and induce paralysis of one or more eye muscles. But you have been warned!

There are a great many products on the market these days which exploit the magical name ginseng. You can find ginseng with chicken broth, ginseng tea and so on. Be warned that these products have no ginseng value to them at all. They are certainly not medicinal. The ginseng in them is minimal and of so poor a quality that you are wasting your money paying for the name.

Eleutherococcus senticosus is available in a number of health stores. It is manufactured in the USSR with the approval of the Soviet government and instructions are usually included on the container. The recommended dose is 20 to 40 drops before meals, repeated 2 or 3 times a day to not more than 80 drops a day, in a little water. For children, one drop per year of age, twice a day. A full course of treatment lasts for 25 to 30 days. Rest for one or two weeks and repeat again if you wish to.

CHAPTER EIGHT
The Cultivation of Ginseng

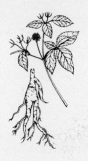

It is hard to find the ginseng plant in the wild, whether in the wilds of America or the most remote parts of China and Siberia. It is a somewhat reclusive plant, with a particular liking for shady forested slopes where it can spread its succulent roots far in search of water and nutriments. It takes several years to mature, usually producing no seeds until it is well into its third year of growth. By this time, it is anything from five to nine inches high. In its third year, the plant flowers, producing greenish yellow blossoms which develop into berries. It is these scarlet berries which draw attention to the plant in the autumn. They each contain seeds— one, two or three in number—from which new plants will develop. Each year from the third year onwards, the plant shoots up, flowers and seeds, and then the foliage falls away, leaving a small scar on the main stem. The number of these scars gives the age of the plant.

With ginseng bringing in the prices that it does, it has obviously not been left to nature to take care of its production. The growing of ginseng is a skilled task and the Koreans have taken its mastery further than most. They have probably had the longest practice in doing so: Korean records claim a history of 5,000 years of cultivation of the plant.

The plant grows best in well-drained sandy loam or clay with a high content of potassium. No chemical fertilisers are used, but certain crops are considered to prepare the soil best for the ginseng planting: wheat, barley, soybeans, sweet potatoes and upland rice. The soil content is so important because ginseng is a slow-growing plant. The beds are all north or north-east facing.

The seeds for the nursery plants are gathered in July from four-year-old plants. After the berries are plucked from the plants, the seeds are removed, washed and dried so as to encourage the opening of the seed hulls. The seeds are sown in early November and they are then tended in the nursery beds until they are from 15 to 17 months old. At this point, they are transplanted to their permanent beds and the roots are harvested anything from three to five years later. The best harvest time for white ginseng is between July and August and for the red between August and October.

The two colours do not refer to different types of ginseng but merely to differences in their processing. White ginseng is made by peeling off the outer skin and drying the root in the sun. Red ginseng is made by steaming the raw ginseng and then drying it artificially in a heated room. In Korea, anyone may grow and process white ginseng, but the Korean governments—both North and South—control the production of red ginseng. This is presumably because it is such a major feature in the overseas earnings of both countries that they cannot afford the kind of scandal that has hit the Italian wine trade in recent years.

After processing, the roots are sorted carefully into various grades, determined by the thickness and fullness of the roots. The Korean government grading tables run as follows: the best grade is known as Heaven, the next as Earth, Good is third and Tails is fourth. The grade known as Tails is mainly used for the making of teas and other ginseng preparations where quality is not important. The roots are finally sold by weight, in approximately one-pound packages either wholesale to overseas merchants or through the thousands of direct-outlet Korean emporia all over the world.

Do not think of growing your own ginseng. Even if you wished to go through the process and could get hold of active seeds, it is unlikely to be successful .

CHAPTER NINE

Buying Ginseng

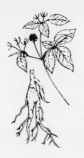

The commercial value of ginseng is such that it is well worth the ingenious and unprincipled retailer trying his luck on the unwary with counterfeit goods. Even experts sometimes have a problem with roots treated cunningly enough, so do not think that you are going to do better.

No public scandal has ever been attached to the Korean direct-selling emporia—no scandal about the quality of their produce, anyway. There have been suggestions that some of the emporia might have been a cover for other activities, sometimes of a political nature, but that need not be your concern. Since Korean ginseng is graded strictly and sold according to grading, it should be an easy matter to purchase the root of the quality you can afford.

When it comes to other ginseng dealers, this may not always be so. It is better therefore to deal only with herbalists you consider trustworthy and reliable, as well as knowledgeable. A Chinese traditional herbalist would be such a person, if you have established a good relationship. Other herbalists and health food stores are now beginning to deal in ginseng but most of them could not be considered experts in selection of the plant nor, perhaps, experts in the right storage of the root.

When it comes to Eleuthero, it is already packaged into liquid and processed for use as drops, so there is little need to worry about what you are getting. You are buying a standardised processed tonic.

American ginseng is sold usually through Chinese herbal stores and you could probably get it through such outlets in the major cities. It is not sorted and graded in the same way as *Ginseng panax* and its price should reflect that.

Just remember that there are no bargains in ginseng. If it is cheap, it is bad or spurious. If it is tea, soup, or some other ginseng-labelled product, forget it. You are paying for the name of a substance which is only barely present in the product.

CHAPTER TEN

Directory of Ginseng

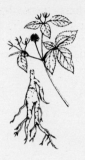

Watch out for ginseng with vague labelling, like Manchurian ginseng or Asiatic ginseng. These terms mean nothing in the grading accepted by Korean and Chinese herbal dealers. When such products have been tested for active ingredients, they have come out low and you will probably be wasting your money. Look for *Ginseng panax*, *Ginseng panax*-CA Meyer, Korean panax-CA Meyer and specific listings of that kind.

LONDON
Korean Ginseng Centre
Charing Cross Road
London W1
Tel: 01-240–0636
A central supply place for ginseng, which can also be ordered by mail. Korean ginseng prices are fixed and therefore you can get an idea of what you should be paying for quality root.

Check your *Yellow Pages* for Chinese herbalists in your area. There are such herbalists in all major cities throughout Britain, serving mainly the local Chinese community. However, these days, they are also accustomed to inquisitive westerners and will probably be helpful. They will certainly have all kinds of grades of ginseng and can offer you a variety of roots.

Additionally, there are a number of health food and herbal stores which stock Korean ginseng tablets, usually described as Korean red kooga. While no respectable Chinese would be caught buying tablets when the root is available, these have been tested and found to contain chemically active ingredients, like the roots. It is second best but would meet many people's wishes. Some reliable stockists of Korean red ginseng tablets are:

The Midnight Shop
223 Brompton Road
London SW3
Tel: 01-589–5030
Open Monday to Sunday, 10 a.m. to midnight

Holland & Barrett
(11 branches all over London)

Outside London, the major cities usually have a Korean Ginseng Centre (check the telephone book) from which roots can be bought. Other shops offering red ginseng tablets are:

The Happy Nut House
183 Princess Pavement
Birkenhead
Merseyside
Tel: 051-647–6361
Will order what you want with an agreed minimum.

CNS Moorey Herbs and Health Foods
41 Salford Road
Blackburn
Lancashire
Tel: 0254-53245
Will obtain and mail what you want.

English Grain Ltd
Swains Park Road
Overseal
Burton-on-Trent
Staffordshire
Tel: 0283–221616

Life & Health Foods
Fifers Lane Trading Estate
Norwich
Stock some ginseng roots, including red and white.

Sources

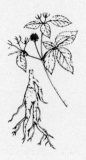

All the traditional Chinese medical information about ginseng was supplied by fourth-generation Chinese healer, Dr Gary Chak-kei Butt.

The scientific, chemical and biochemical information about current exploration and experimentation with ginseng was supplied by the biochemists, botanists, biologists and chemists of the Chinese University's World Health Organisation Project investigating the properties of ginseng.

Information about types, growing and choosing of ginseng comes from Kwan Pak-cheung, the world's biggest dealer in ginseng.

Additional source material included the following:
Li Shih-chen, *Pen Tsao Kang Mu*, trans. 1874 by Drs Smith and Stuart.
Polo, Marco, *Travels*, 1294, Penguin edition.
Pen Tsao, published in China, c. AD 200 (material translated by G Butt).
Royal Society of London, 1714, Father Jartroux's report to the Vatican (1711); *Eleutherococcus*, 1968.
Vogel, Virgil, *American Indian Medicine*, University of Oklahoma Press, 1970.

Information on scientific discoveries about ginseng comes from Dr Paul But, considered to be one of the world's authorities on ginseng and based at the Chinese University of Hong Kong.

Index